Let's Sleep Together

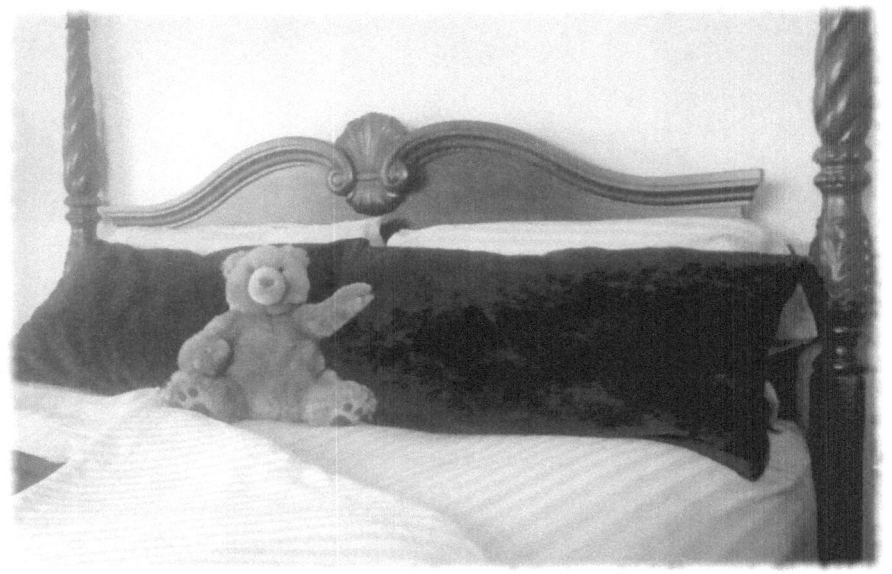

The Bedside Companion

To Knock Yourself Out.

Dennis M. Loreman

ISBN: 1468157833
ISBN-13: 978-1468157833

DEDICATION

I dedicate this book to all my friends. Will you please follow the simple directions in this book and go to sleep right now?!? I wrote this book for you. It is my hope that you will stop complaining about how you are always so tired every time we talk.

Seriously, we all have challenges. Go ahead and sleep on it.

Allow your subconscious to give you some added perspective.

Now, go to sleep!

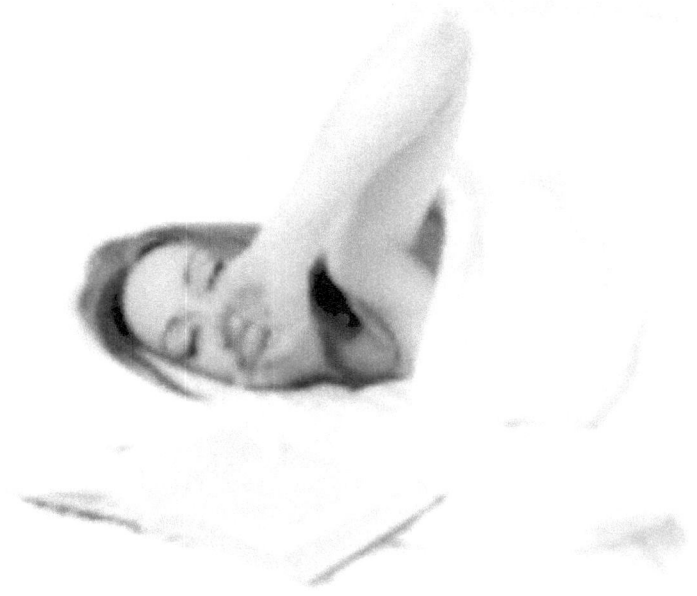

ACKNOWLEDGMENTS

I would like to thank the National Guild of Hypnotists for being a positive, guiding force in helping people make improvements from within themselves.

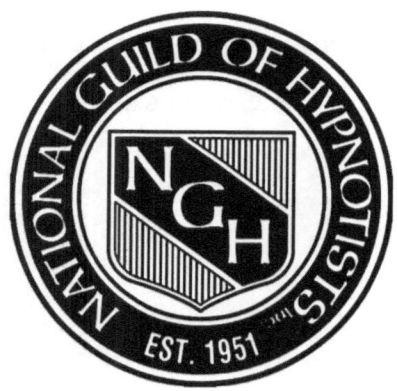

CONTENTS

Introduction

Maybe you are tossing and turning uncomfortably...

Maybe you are thinking about some noise you heard...

Maybe you are concerned about what happened in the past...

Maybe you are contemplating how to handle the next events in your life...

Well, stop it and read on.

This is not a treatise on how to better understand or resolve your life's challenges internally or externally. This book contains no known sedatives that if you lick the pages or your e-reader will cause you to sleep. (Future product is pending regulatory approval.)

What you are reading now is a specialized form of hypnotic writing designed to set your mind, emotions, and body into a well-deserved state of relaxation. These simple techniques have been tested and have turned the worst kind of tossers into the best kind of sleepers.

As long as you can follow the simple and easy exercises described in the text and pictures you'll soon find this book will be a trusted companion ready to sleep with you whenever you want or need it.

Caution: Do not read this book while operating a moving vehicle, cooking a meal, or supervising animals/children/co-workers. The author takes no responsibility for your lack of heed and your complete loss of consciousness.

Please sleep responsibly.

Now, let's sleep together.

Purpose

Can you imagine a time when you were so very tired that no matter how hard you wanted to not fall deeply asleep you could not keep your eyelids from feeling heavier and heavier until eventually they slipped slowly and softly over your weary eyes? You can now give yourself the permission to let such a feeling settle within you.

Pay no attention to the length of time you have available to sleep and what time you may actually sleep. Studies have shown our perception of time is relative. By following along, a few minutes can be as restful as an hour, and a few hours can be as restful as you need.

The following pages are going to guide you through simple patterns to bring you closer and closer to closing your eyes and putting your body and mind at rest.

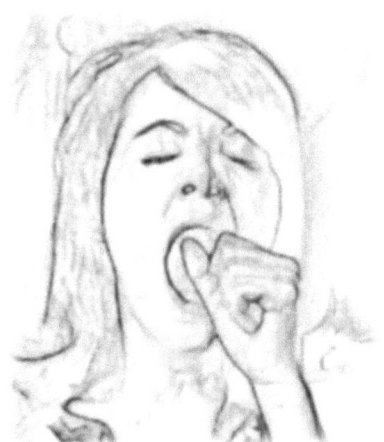

Now as you see the picture of the person yawning, feel the yawning sensation build within you and start to relax you.

Alarms

Physical:

If you have a planned event in the future and you need to rise at a certain time, be sure to properly set an alarm to provide ample time to prepare.

Mental:

If you do not have an alarm, do not trust your alarm, or do not trust you will wake up with your alarm, then see the classic alarm image below. Imagine the hands of the clock indicating the time you want to awake.

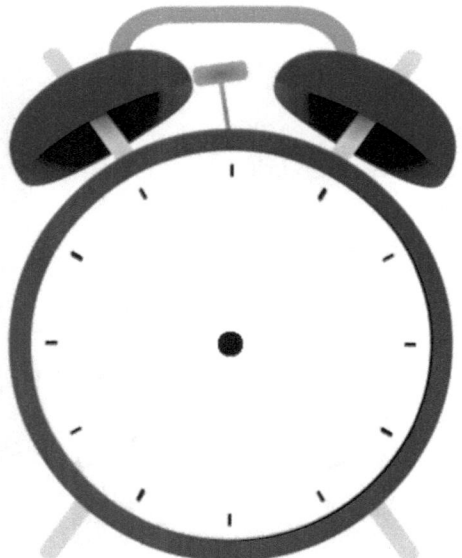

Now close your eyes for just a moment and see the hands of the clock indicating the time you want to awake. You may also imagine a digital clock reading the time you need to awake as well.

Say in your mind or aloud, "I want to awake at ____ as it is important to me, but until then I allow myself to let time pass as I sleep."

Environment Check

Take just a brief moment to look around wherever you decided to rest and make any changes around your sleeping area to reduce the chance of being disturbed unnecessarily. Unless you have already used the restroom or have no need of such facilities, then now is the best moment to put down this book and take care of yourself.

Ease your mind in knowing that while you may fall into a deep sleep, if there was an emergency; know your subconscious will wake you, as without your physical body it would have no home.

Now allow yourself to move into the most comfortable position for sleeping.

From this moment forward any sounds you may hear such as weather, traffic, or other persons will just pass by you. Any sounds will pass over you like water over a rock in a stream and will only help you settle deeper into relaxation and sleep.

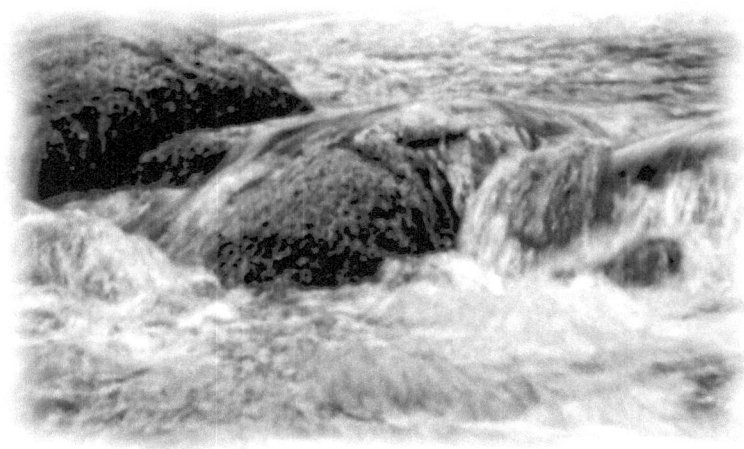

Issue Box

Review Your Thoughts

This image below is a box where you will imagine any and all of your concerns and place them for just the time you need to rest. Placing your concerns in the box will give you a chance to be free from thoughts or worries so you may rest peacefully.

Imagine tracing the X for each concern to let it pass from your mind to dwell in the box. Allow each concern to be securely placed here, so it may be dealt with at a later time after you have rested. If you are inclined, it may help naming the concern as you trace it thereby reinforcing its placement in the box.

Example:

"I place this concern over my job/health/family/friend into this box".

Lock Your Box

See the box is now closed and sealed with your special lock.

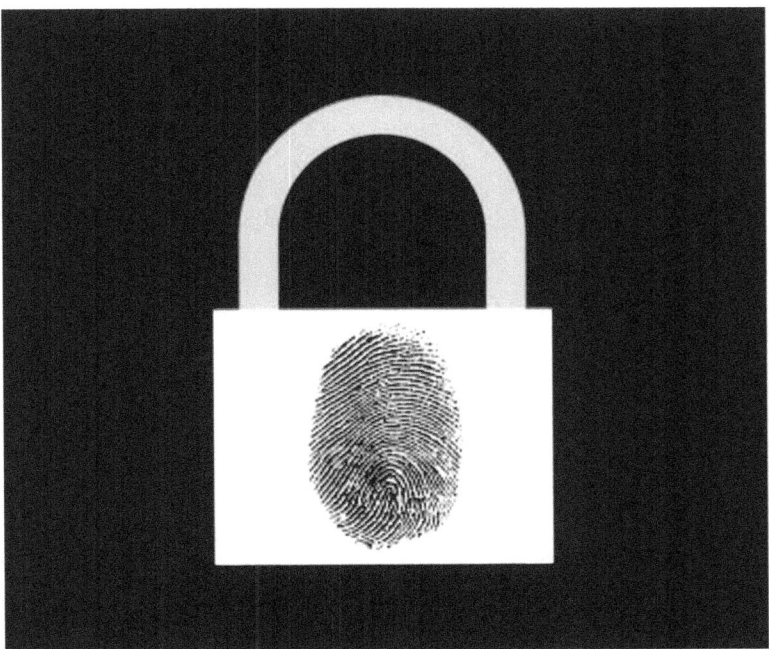

All concerns will stay in this box allowing you to rest peacefully. You can now narrow your focus on relaxation and falling deeply asleep.

If any further concerns arise, you may imagine the open box or turn back to the open box image and place it inside the box and then close and re-seal the box.

Physical Relaxation

The following progressive relaxation pattern will allow your body to carry you into your dreams as easily as, if not better than, it carries you while awake.

You will focus on a small part of your body and tense each part during a deep inhalation and then relax that part with a long exhalation. If you find it difficult to tense certain parts of your body or have limitations that prevent the physical act of tensing, simply imagine tensing and relaxing the body part.

While tensing, imagine the perfect physical and healthy embodiment of the region settling inside that part of you during the relaxation.

Deep breaths will be most relaxing through the nose when possible and filling the bottom of your lungs first to extend your diaphragm. After holding for just a few moments, release the air back out through your nose.

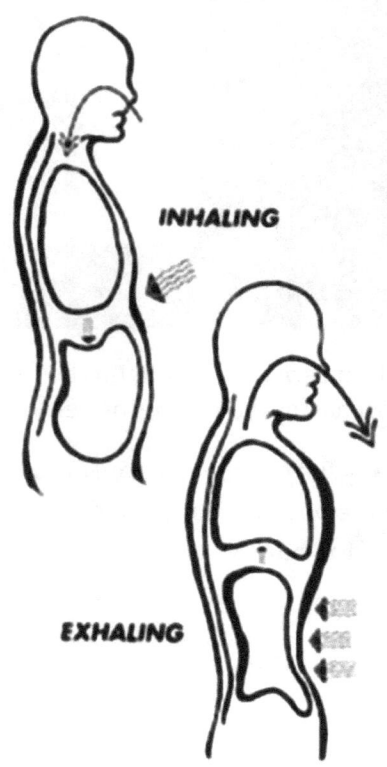

INHALING

If you are inclined to verbalize while you exhale, allow the word "Me" to be drawn out ('Mmmmeeeeeeee') as the mental attention mixes with the physical air passing through your body.

Now, take 3 deep breaths with your attention on just inhaling and exhaling through your nose and then start on your body...

EXHALING

Toes

See the image below and notice the area highlights the toes.

Place your focus on your toes.

Take a deep inhalation and clench your toes at the same time and hold for a few moments.

Imagine them in perfect physical health.

Exhale slowly and relax your toes at the same time.

Allow them to be completely at peace and in a state of restfulness.

Repeat another deep breath with your attention on your toes until you feel they are resting and then slip to the next body part.

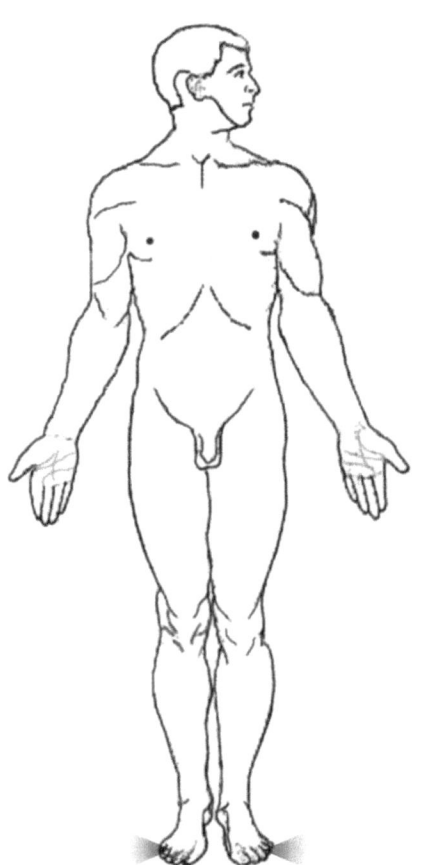

Feet

See the image below and notice the area highlights the feet.

Place your focus on your feet.

Take a deep inhalation and tense your feet at the same time and hold for a few moments.

Imagine them in perfect physical health.

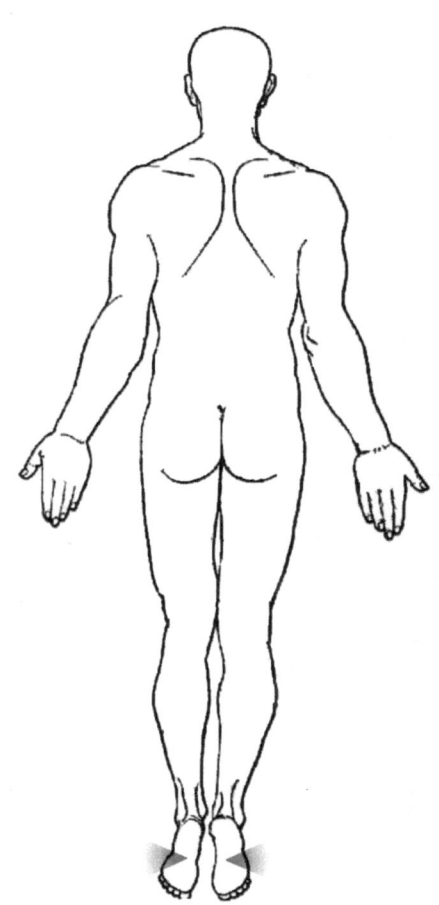

Exhale slowly and relax your feet at the same time.

Allow them to be completely at peace and in a state of restfulness.

Repeat another deep breath with your attention on your feet until you feel they are resting and then slip to the next body part.

Ankles

See the image below and notice the area highlights the ankles.

Place your focus on your ankles.

Take a deep inhalation and tense your ankles to extend your toes at the same time and hold for a few moments.

Imagine them in perfect physical health.

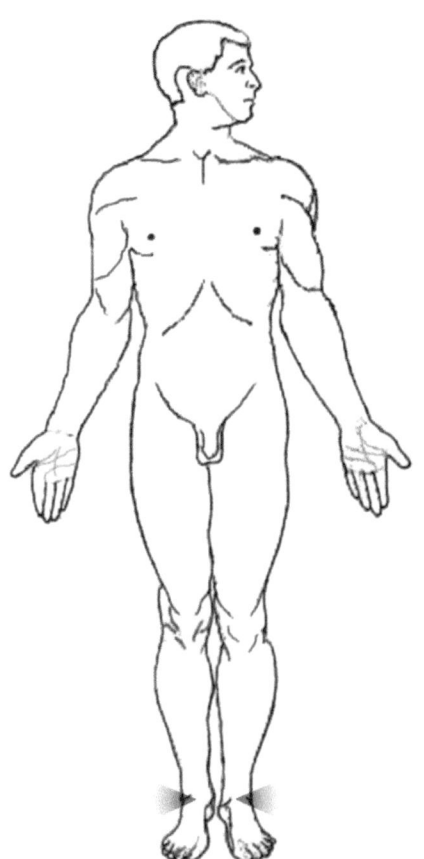

Exhale slowly and relax your ankles at the same time.

Allow them to be completely at peace and in a state of restfulness.

Repeat another deep breath with your attention on your ankles until you feel they are resting and then slip to the next body part.

Calves

See the image below and notice the area highlights the calves.

Place your focus on your calves.

Take a deep inhalation and tense your calves at the same time and hold for a few moments.

Imagine them in perfect physical health.

Exhale slowly and relax your calves at the same time.

Allow them to be completely at peace and in a state of restfulness.

Repeat another deep breath with your attention on your calves until you feel they are resting and then slip to the next body part.

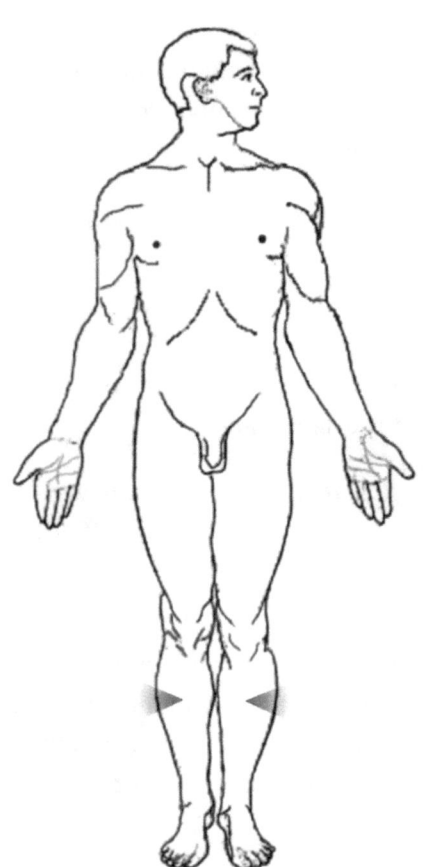

Knees

See the image below and notice the area highlights the knees.

Place your focus on your knees.

Take a deep inhalation and tense your knees to extend your legs at the same time and hold for a few moments.

Imagine them in perfect physical health.

Exhale slowly and relax your knees at the same time.

Allow them to be completely at peace and in a state of restfulness.

Repeat another deep breath with your attention on your knees until you feel they are resting and then slip to the next body part.

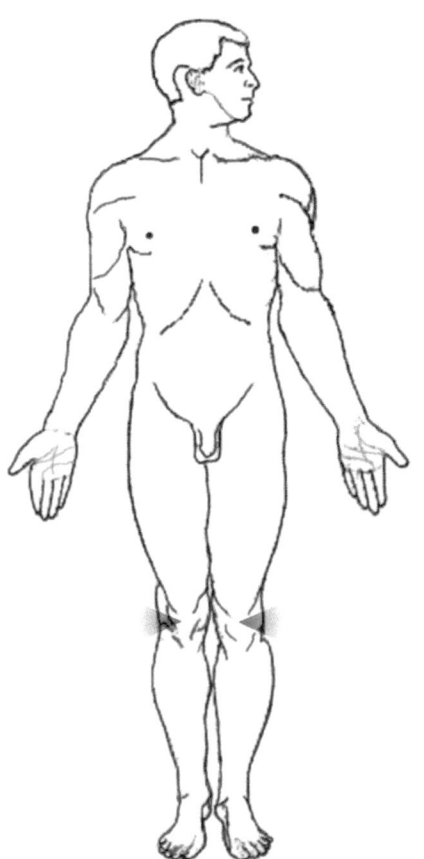

Thighs

See the image below and notice the area highlights the thighs.

Place your focus on your thighs.

Take a deep inhalation and tense your thighs at the same time and hold for a few moments.

Imagine them in perfect physical health.

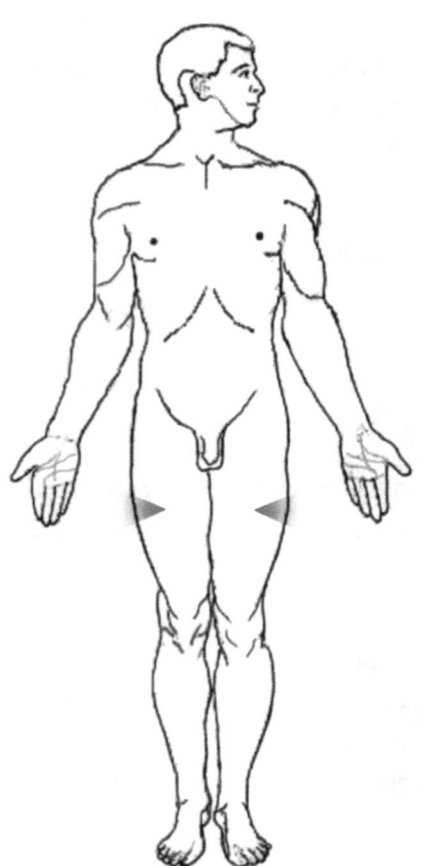

Exhale slowly and relax your thighs at the same time.

Allow them to be completely at peace and in a state of restfulness.

Repeat another deep breath with your attention on your thighs until you feel they are resting and then slip to the next body part.

Bottom

See the image below and notice the area highlights the bottom (buttocks).

Place your focus on your bottom.

Take a deep inhalation and tense your bottom at the same time and hold for a few moments.

Imagine this part of you in perfect physical health.

Exhale slowly and relax your bottom at the same time.

Allow this part of you to be completely at peace and in a state of restfulness.

Repeat another deep breath with your attention on your bottom until you feel it is resting and then slip to the next body part.

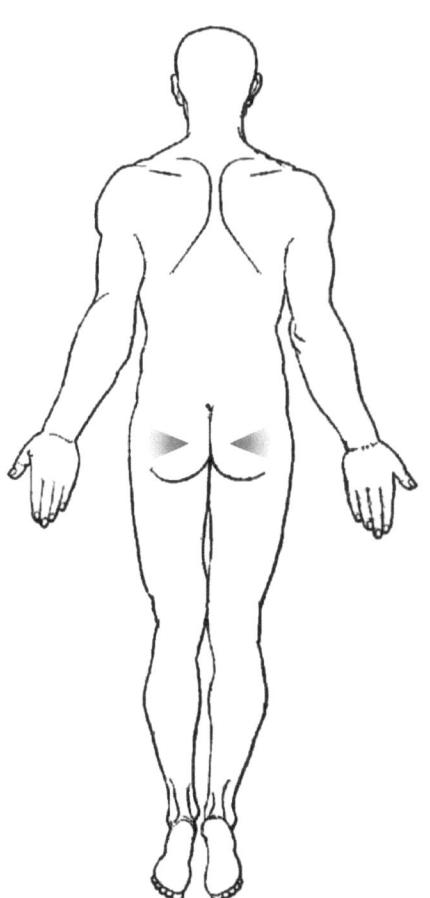

Genitalia

See the image below and notice the area highlights the genitals.

Place your focus on your genitalia.

Take a deep inhalation and tense your genitalia (perineum) at the same time and hold for a few moments.

Imagine this part of you in perfect physical health.

Exhale slowly and relax your genitalia at the same time.

Allow this part of you to be completely at peace and in a state of restfulness.

Repeat another deep breath with your attention on your genitalia until you feel it is resting and then slip to the next body part.

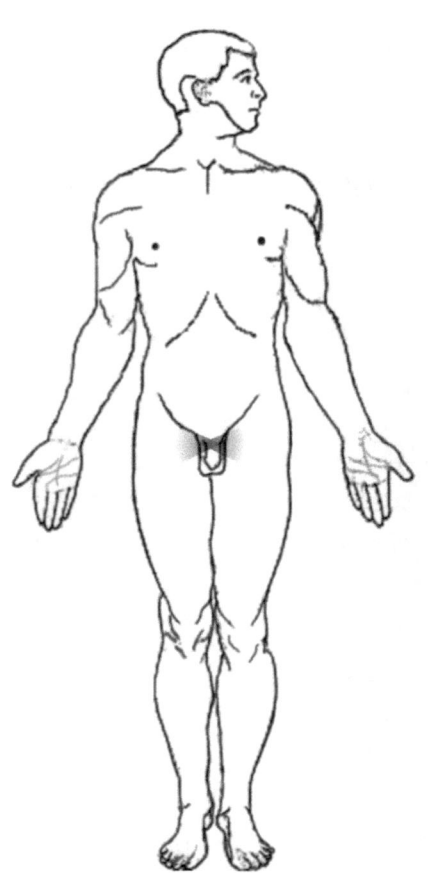

Abdomen

See the image below and notice the area highlights the abdomen.

Place your focus on your abdomen.

Take a deep inhalation and tense your abdomen (stomach muscles) at the same time and hold for a few moments.

Imagine this part of you in perfect physical health.

Exhale slowly and relax your abdomen at the same time.

Allow this part of you to be completely at peace and in a state of restfulness.

Repeat another deep breath with your attention on your abdomen until you feel it is resting and then slip to the next body part.

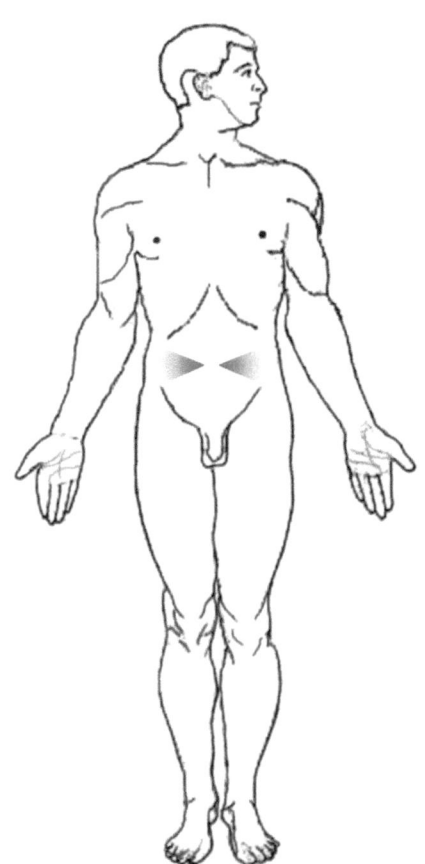

Heart

See the image below and notice the area highlights the heart.

Place your focus on your heart.

Take a deep inhalation and focus on your heart beating and the circulation of your blood all at the same time for a few moments.

Imagine this part of you in perfect physical health.

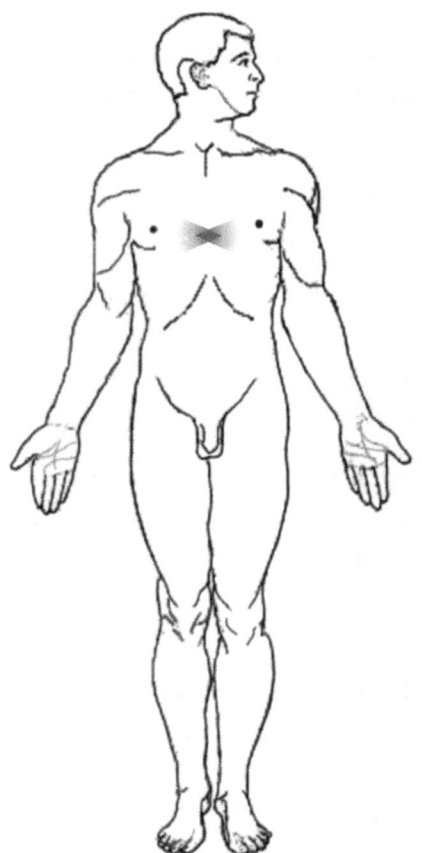

Exhale slowly and allow the focus on your heart to relax at the same time.

Allow this part of you to be completely at peace and in a state of restfulness.

Repeat another deep breath with your attention on your heart until you feel it is resting and then slip to the next body part.

Lungs

See the image below and notice the area highlights the lungs.

Place your focus on your lungs.

Take a deep inhalation and focus on your lungs and the flow of air deep into them all at the same time and hold for a few moments.

Imagine them in perfect physical health.

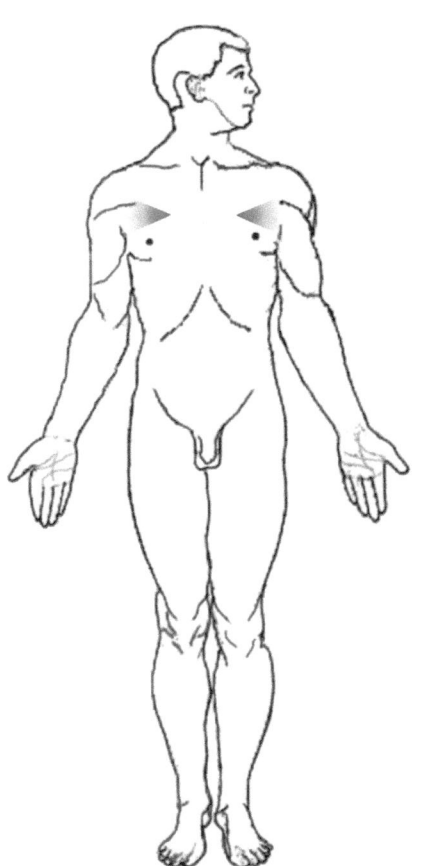

Exhale slowly and allow the focus on your lungs to relax at the same time.

Allow them to be completely at peace and in a state of restfulness.

Repeat another deep breath with your attention on your lungs until you feel they are resting and then slip to the next body part.

Shoulders

See the image below and notice the area highlights the shoulders.

Place your focus on your shoulders.

Take a deep inhalation and tense your shoulders by bringing them up to your neck at the same time and hold for a few moments.

Imagine them in perfect physical health.

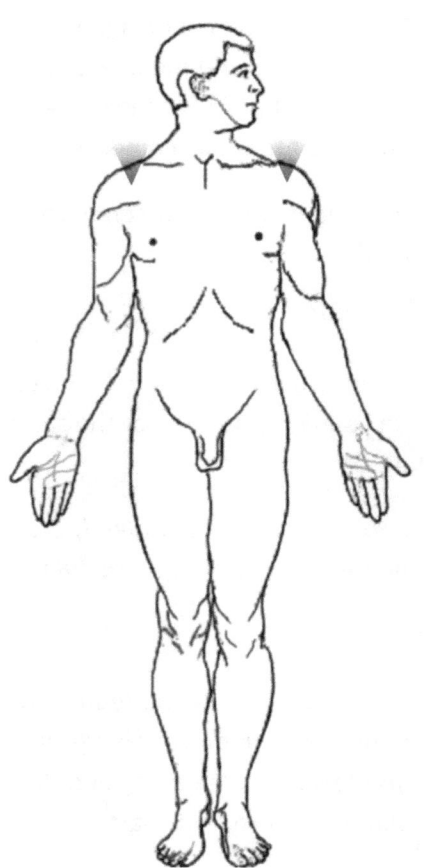

Exhale slowly and relax your shoulders at the same time.

Allow them to be completely at peace and in a state of restfulness.

Repeat another deep breath with your attention on your shoulders until you feel they are resting and then slip to the next body part.

Upper Arms

See the image below and notice the area highlights the upper arms.

Place your focus on your upper arms.

Take a deep inhalation and tense your upper arms at the same time and hold for a few moments.

Imagine them in perfect physical health.

Exhale slowly and relax your upper arms at the same time.

Allow them to be completely at peace and in a state of restfulness.

Repeat another deep breath with your attention on your upper arms until you feel they are resting and then slip to the next body part.

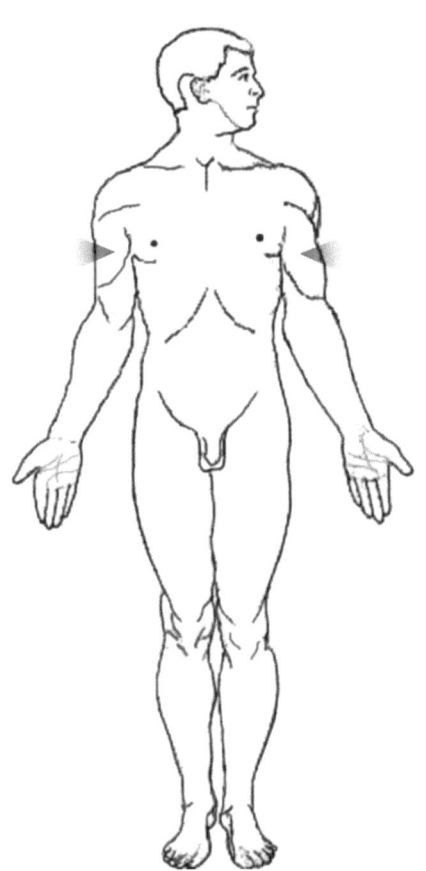

Lower Arms

See the image below and notice the area highlights the lower arms.

Place your focus on your lower arms.

Take a deep inhalation and tense your lower arms at the same time and hold for a few moments.

Imagine them in perfect physical health.

Exhale slowly and relax your lower arms at the same time.

Allow them to be completely at peace and in a state of restfulness.

Repeat another deep breath with your attention on your lower arms until you feel they are resting and then slip to the next body part.

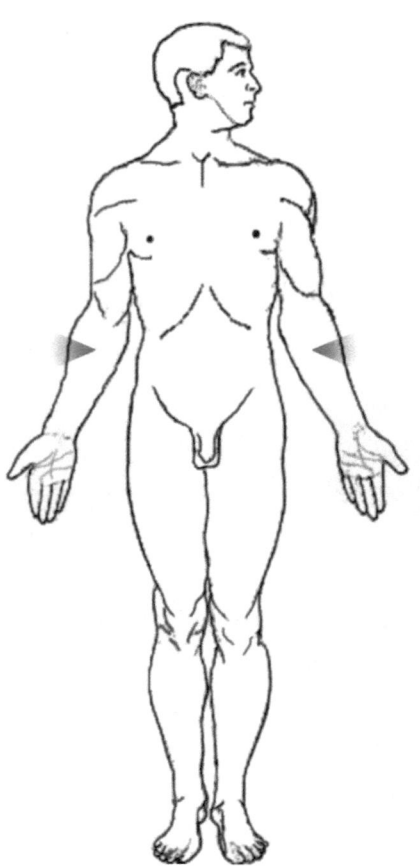

Hands

See the image below and notice the area highlights the hands. You may put the book down while you perform this exercise with your hands.

Place your focus on your hands.

Take a deep inhalation and tense your hands into a tight fist at the same time and hold for a few moments.

Imagine them in perfect physical health.

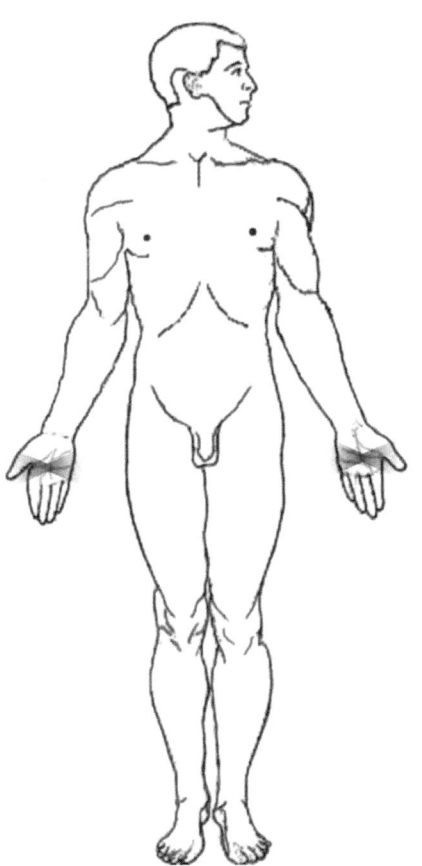

Exhale slowly and relax your hands at the same time.

Allow them to be completely at peace and in a state of restfulness.

Repeat another deep breath with your attention on your hands until you feel they are resting and then slip to the next body part.

Spine

See the image below and notice the area highlights the spine.

Place your focus on your spine.

Take a deep inhalation and focus on your spine as you stretch to lengthen it at the same time and hold for a few moments.

Imagine this part of you in perfect physical health.

Exhale slowly and relax your spine at the same time.

Allow this part of you to be completely at peace and in a state of restfulness.

Repeat another deep breath with your attention on your spine until you feel it is resting and then slip to the next body part.

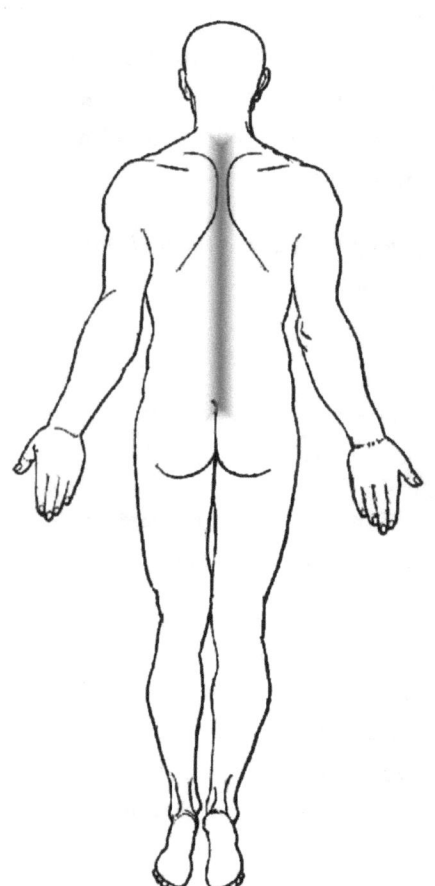

Neck

See the image below and notice the area highlights the neck.

Place your focus on your neck.

Take a deep inhalation and tense your neck as you bring your chin close to your chest at the same time and hold for a few moments.

Imagine this part of you in perfect physical health.

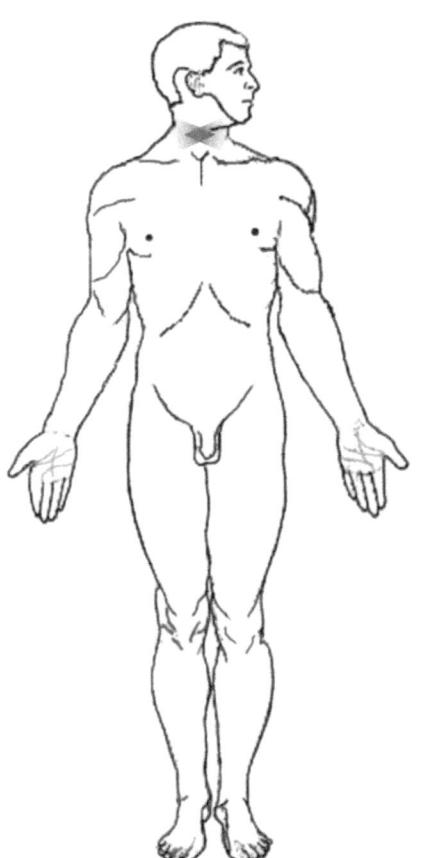

Exhale slowly and relax your neck at the same time.

Allow this part of you to be completely at peace and in a state of restfulness.

Repeat another deep breath with your attention on your neck until you feel it is resting and then slip to the next body part.

Jaw

See the image below and notice the area highlights the jaw.

Place your focus on your jaw.

Take a deep inhalation and tense your jaw as you clench your teeth at the same time and hold for a few moments.

Imagine this part of you in perfect physical health.

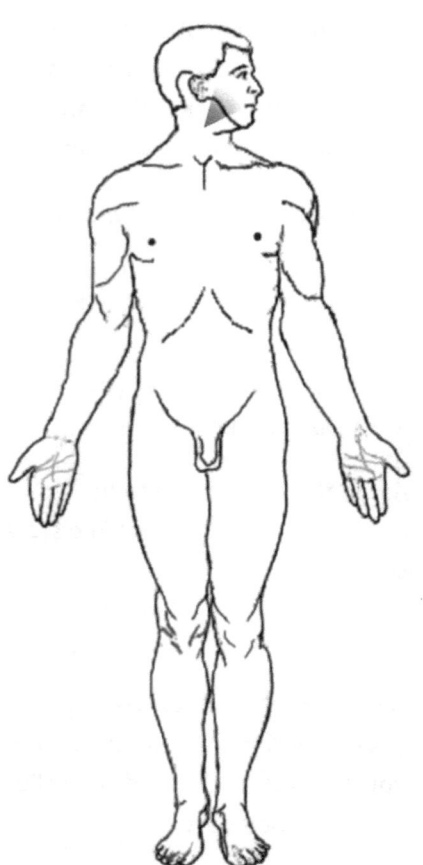

Exhale slowly and relax your jaw at the same time.

Allow this part of you to be completely at peace and in a state of restfulness.

Repeat another deep breath with your attention on your jaw until you feel it is resting and then slip to the next body part.

Forehead

See the image below and notice the area highlights the forehead.

Place your focus on your forehead.

Take a deep inhalation and tense your forehead by squeezing your eyebrows together at the same time and hold for a few moments.

Imagine this part of you in perfect physical health.

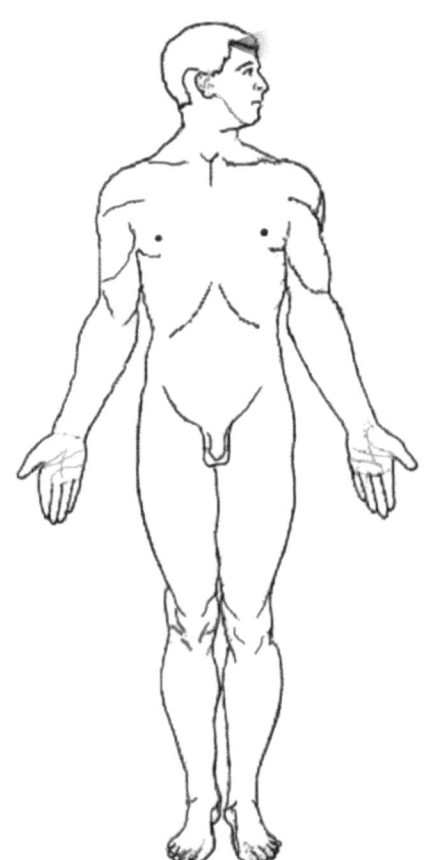

Exhale slowly and relax your forehead at the same time.

Allow this part of you to be completely at peace and in a state of restfulness.

Repeat another deep breath with your attention on your forehead until you feel it is resting and then slip to the next body part.

Eyes

See the image below and notice the area highlights the eyes. By this moment, you may be so comfortable and relaxed that when you relax and close your eyes after tensing them they may stay closed and you just fall asleep. You can allow yourself to go sleep.

Place your focus on your eyes.

Take a deep inhalation and tense your eyes by squeezing your eyes tightly closed at the same time and hold for a few moments.

Imagine them in perfect physical health.

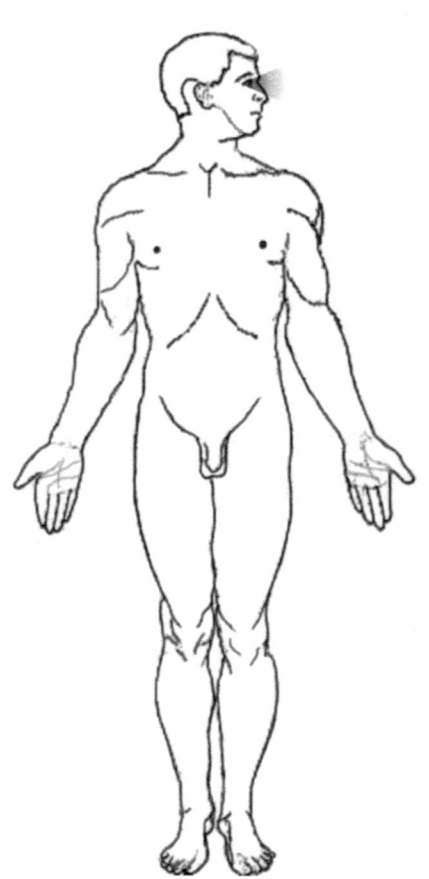

Exhale slowly and relax your eyes at the same time.

Allow them to be completely at peace and in a state of restfulness.

Repeat another deep breath with your attention on your eyes until you feel they are resting and then....

Whole body

See the image below and notice the area highlights the whole body.

Place your focus on your whole body.

Take a deep inhalation and tense your whole body at the same time and hold for a few moments.

Imagine yourself in perfect physical health.

Exhale slowly and relax your whole body at the same time.

Allow yourself to be completely at peace and in a state of restfulness.

Repeat another deep breath with your attention on your whole body until you feel it is resting peacefully.

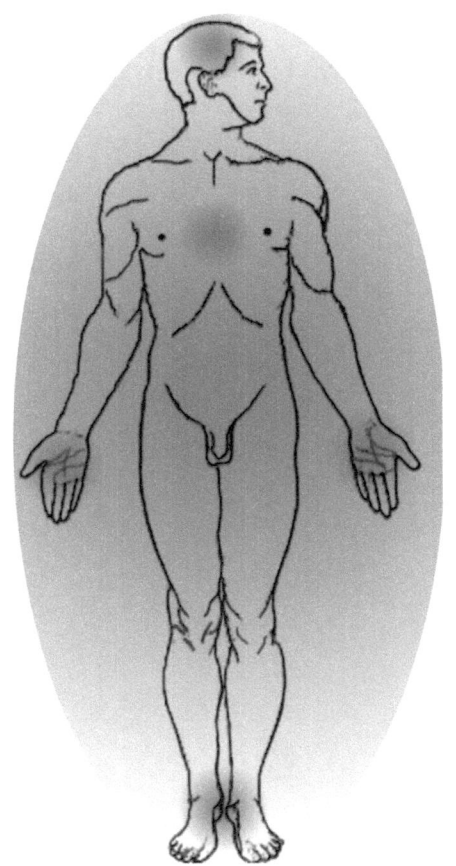

Mental Blanket

Now imagine being wrapped in a warm, golden blanket of peace, comfort, and security as it is placed around your shoulders, neck, and down your whole body.

The warm blanket sensation melts into your body and infuses you with all those qualities to have a restful sleep.

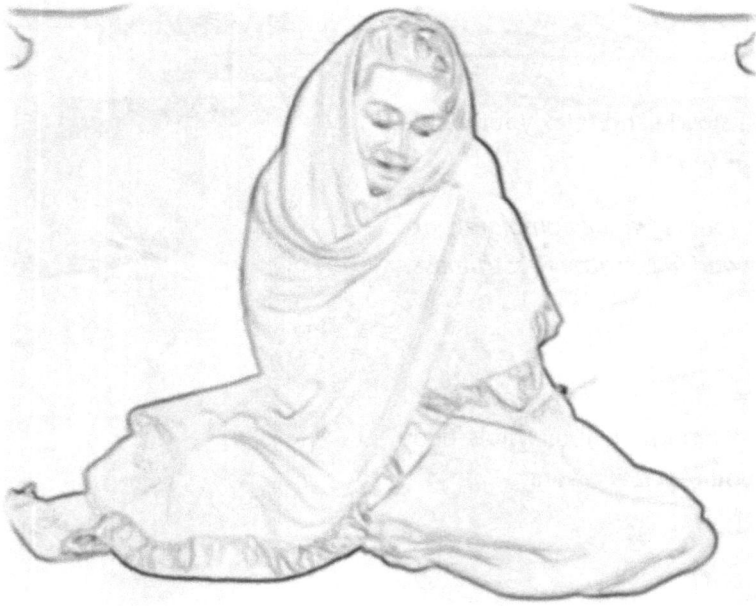

Tired Eyes and Closing Book

See the image below and allow your eyes to slowly trace the loops of the spiral from the outside to the inside and then inside to the outside repeatedly.

When you see a "zzz" at the top of a loop in the spiral, within the silent chamber of your mind say, "*Deep, deep sleep; sleep, sleep deep*". With each loop of the spiral your eyes will feel more and more tired, weary, and heavy until they close for sleep.

You may close the book at anytime and its closing will carry you into a deep restful sleep. You may still see the spiral in your mind as you fall deeply asleep.

"Deep, deep sleep; sleep, sleep deep"

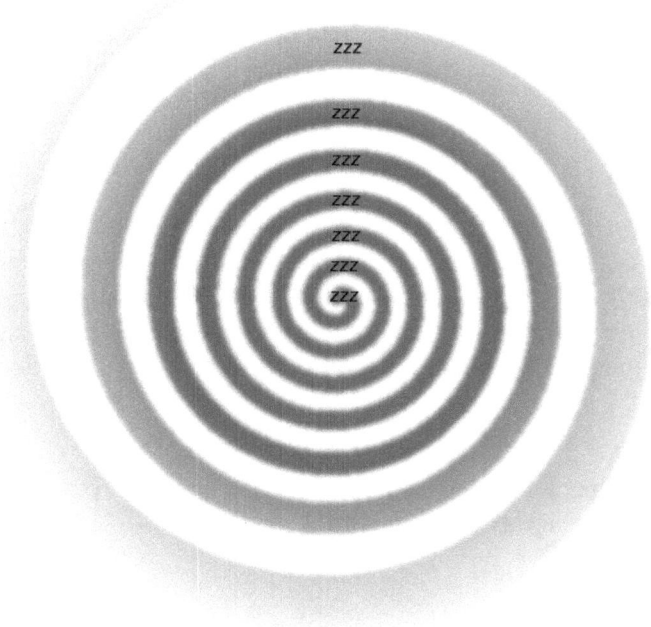

Considerations

If you are still reading and have not fallen asleep yet, return to the previous page and follow the pattern and instructions closely.

If you have just woken from a restful sleep, no matter how long, congratulations on your making the most of this book.

After you have rested, remember to unlock your issues box and follow-up on your loose ends. You will feel much better for such accomplishments and you will spend less time placing concerns in the box when you repeat that section.

Although all pages from the Purpose section to the Tired Eyes section are important, you may find that after a few times of following the exercises in this book, just reviewing the spiral diagram will allow you to quickly and easily fall asleep.

You may be surprised at how easily this book can help you sleep, not just by yourself, but also with a friend. For the friends you do not want to sleep with, but want to move beyond the lack of sleep issue in your everyday conversations, this book can be very beneficial to you and them. Please recommend this book or just purchase a copy for such friends.

Thank you for taking the time to sleep with this book and may your restful periods come as quick as you need them.

About the Author

Dennis Loreman has been a certified hypnotherapist for over a decade and has helped many people suffering from a variety of issues find peace and resolution. He is an exploratory hypnotist advancing techniques and approaches that stretch the boundaries of human consciousness and its perceived limits.

"Whether it's a short nap or long sleep, some of life's best solutions come from those restful moments inside a dreamscape."

Other works by the Author:

You are Getting Very Sleepy: Guided Hypnosis for Sleeping

Audio CD: https://www.createspace.com/1717018

Mind the Road: Waking Hypnosis for a Conscious Commute

Audio CD: https://www.createspace.com/1713709

These works are also available on Amazon.com.

www.ingramcontent.com/pod-product-compliance
Lightning Source LLC
Chambersburg PA
CBHW061232280526
45784CB00006B/2736